Special Mediterranean Diet Cookbook

Enjoy your Meal with These Yummy Recipes

Mateo Buscema

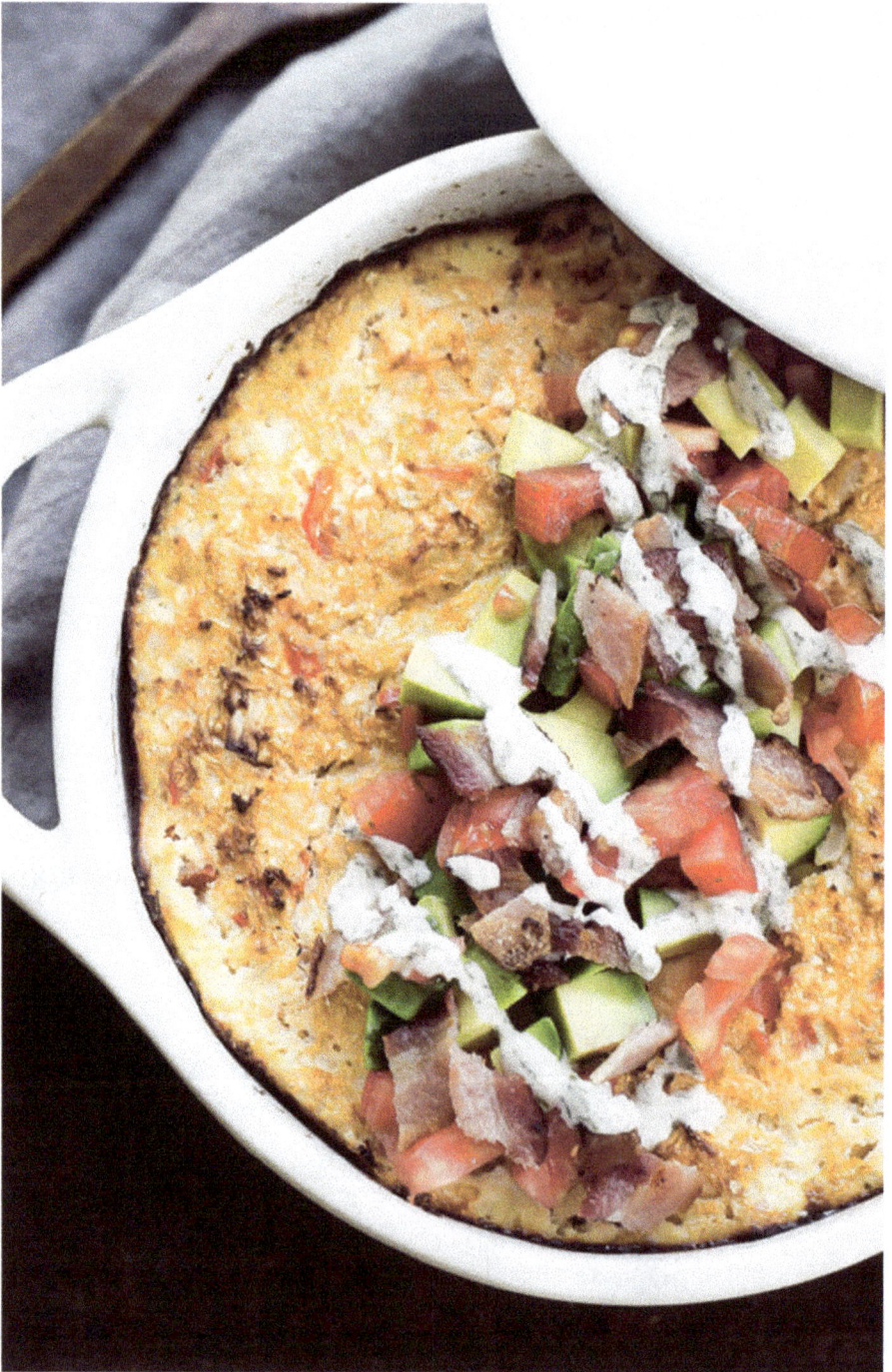

TABLE OF CONTENTS

Easy butternut squash recipe with lentils and quinoa

This recipe is augmented with lentils and quinoa for a satisfying lunch with Mediterranean diet spices an extra crunch derived from roasted almonds and warm fall salad.

Ingredients

- Large handful of fresh parsley, chopped
- 1 whole butternut squash
- Salt
- 2 teaspoons of allspice , divided
- ½ cup of toasted slivered almonds
- Fresh lemon juice
- 1 teaspoon of coriander , divided
- 1 teaspoon of paprika , divided
- 6 garlic cloves, peeled
- Private reserve extra virgin olive oil
- 1 cup of dry quinoa
- 1 cup of dry black lentils, sorted and rinsed
- Water
- 2 scallions, white and green parts, trimmed and chopped

- ¾ teaspoon of cumin
- 2 teaspoons of ground cinnamon, divided

Directions

1. Preheat oven to 425°F.
2. Microwave butternut squash for 3 minutes.
3. Place cubed butternut squash on a large baking sheet.
4. Season with salt.
5. Sprinkle with cinnamon, allspice, coriander, paprika, and cumin.
6. Drizzle with private reserve extra virgin olive oil and toss.
7. Spread the squash in one layer on the sheet pan.
8. Place on the middle rack of heated oven.
9. When ready fried in 15 minutes, remove and add the garlic cloves and drizzle with a little olive oil. Toss squash cubes.
10. Return to oven for another 10 minutes.
11. Place black lentils in a sauce pan and add 3 cups of water.
12. Season with salt boil.
13. Lower the heat let simmer for 25 minutes.
14. Drain any excess oil.
15. Place rinsed quinoa in another saucepan.
16. Add 2 cups of water.
17. Season with salt, boil, then lower heat let simmer for 20 minutes.

18. Place cooked lentils and quinoa in a large bowl.

19. Season with the remainder of spices and a little salt.

20. Toss a little to combine.

21. Add the cooked butternut squash.

22. Chop the roasted garlic and add together with the scallions and fresh parsley.

23. Toss all the ingredients together.

24. Add fresh lemon juice to your taste

25. Add a generous drizzle of extra virgin olive oil. Toss.

26. Taste and adjust accordingly and top with tomatoes.

27. Serve warm and enjoy.

Vegetarian egg casserole

This is a non-static Mediterranean vegetable recipe. It is versatile, in that you change the veggies according to your liking.

Ingredients

- 4 ounces of artichoke hearts
- 3 ounces of crumbled feta cheese
- 1 ounce of chopped fresh parsley
- ½ teaspoon of baking powder
- Kosher salt and black pepper
- 3 ounces of sliced mushrooms
- 1 bell pepper sliced into rounds
- 1 teaspoon of dry oregano
- 8 large eggs
- 1 teaspoon of sweet paprika
- Extra virgin olive oil
- ¼ teaspoon of nutmeg
- 1 ½ cups of milk
- 3 slices bread cut into ½ inch pieces
- 2 shallots, thinly sliced
- 1 tomato, small diced
- 2 ounces of pitted Kalamata olives, sliced

Directions

1. Start by heating your oven to 375°F.
2. In a large mixing bowl, whisk together the eggs, milk, baking powder, salt, pepper, and spices.
3. Add the bread pieces, artichoke hearts, shallots, mushrooms, tomatoes, Kalamata olives, feta and parsley. Mix.
4. Lightly brush the casserole dish with extra virgin olive oil.
5. Transfer the egg and vegetable mixture into the casserole dish and spread evenly.
6. Organize the bell pepper slices on top.
7. Bake for about 35 to 45 minutes.
8. Let the casserole to settle.
9. Cut through and serve.
10. Enjoy.

Feta and spinach frittata

Ingredients

- 1 teaspoon of dried oregano
- Extra virgin olive oil
- ½ teaspoon of dill weed
- 3 tablespoons of chopped fresh mint leaves
- 3 garlic cloves, minced
- ½ teaspoon of black pepper
- ¼ cup of milk
- 4 ounces of crumbled feta cheese
- 8 eggs
- ½ teaspoon of paprika
- ¼ teaspoon of baking powder
- pinch salt
- 6 ounces of frozen chopped spinach
- ½ cup finely chopped yellow onion
- 1 cup chopped fresh parsley

Directions

1. Preheat your oven to 375°F.
2. In a large bowl, whisk together eggs, spices, baking powder, and pinch of salt.

3. Add spinach and all remaining ingredients to the egg mixture. Mix.
4. In a skillet, heat 2 tablespoons of olive oil until shimmering without smoke.
5. Pour in the egg mixture. shake to allow the egg mixture to spread well.
6. Cook on medium-high heat for 4 minutes.
7. Transfer to heated oven to finish cooking for 8 minutes.
8. Serve and enjoy with 3 ingredient Mediterranean salad.

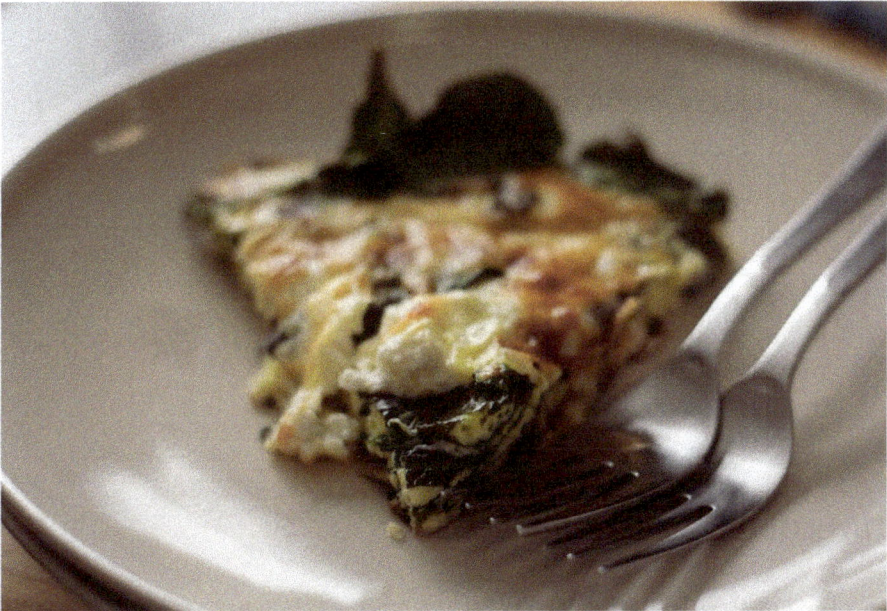

Simple roasted carrots recipe

Do not underestimate these carrots, they need to be roasted over high heat as opposed to low heat otherwise they will take longer than they are supposed to. They get tender and incredibly sweet.

Ingredients

- Parsley for garnish
- ½ lime juice of lemon
- Extra virgin olive oil
- Spices of your choice
- Kosher salt
- 2 lb. carrots peeled and cut on diagonal
- Black pepper
- 1 garlic clove finely minced

Directions

1. Heat your oven to 400°F.
2. Place the sliced carrots in a large mixing bowl, and add a generous drizzle of extra virgin olive oil.
3. Season with kosher salt and black pepper. Toss.
4. Transfer the carrots to a baking pan, spread well in one single layer.

5. Roast in the heated oven for 30 minutes.

6. Turn carrots over to get even color on both sides.

7. Transfer the roasted carrots to a serving bowl.

8. Add flavor to your liking.

9. Season with turmeric and harissa spice blend.

10. If desired, add a little minced garlic and a splash of lime juice.

11. Serve and enjoy.

Pesto pasta recipe with tomatoes and mozzarella

The pesto pasta recipe is a perfect coat for the pasta with sauce to attain a maximum flavor with juicy roasted tomatoes and frozen mozzarella for a perfect Mediterranean diet dinner.

Ingredients

- 6 ounces of fresh baby mozzarella
- 1 cup of basil pesto
- 2 lb.. small tomatoes halved
- Fresh basil for garnish
- Kosher salt and black pepper
- Extra virgin olive oil
- 1 lb.. thin spaghetti
- 2 garlic cloves minced

Directions

1. Start by heating your oven to 450°F.
2. In a larger bowl, toss the tomatoes with kosher salt, black pepper, garlic and extra virgin olive oil.

3. Transfer to a sheet-pan and bake in heated oven for 35 minutes.

4. As the tomatoes roast, cook the spaghetti in boiling water as per the package Directions.

5. Drain any excess water, reserving ½ cup for later.

6. Transfer the cooked spaghetti to a large bowl.

7. Add the pesto and toss to coat.

8. Taste and adjust the seasoning accordingly.

9. Add the roasted tomatoes and mozzarella to the bowl of pasta, toss.

10. Serve and enjoy warm with basil if you desire.

Vegetarian sweet potatoes stew

This is a whole meal fit for breakfast, lunch, and dinner. It is loaded with potatoes with a natural Mediterranean Sea diet sweetness elevated by tomatoes, carrots and silted baby spinach.

Ingredients

- 5 ounces of baby spinach
- 1 teaspoon of ground coriander
- Extra virgin olive oil
- 1 large yellow onion, chopped
- 4 garlic cloves, minced
- 3 carrots, peeled and chopped
- 1 cup of chopped fresh parsley
- 3 sweet potatoes, peeled and cubed
- ¾ teaspoon of Aleppo pepper
- Kosher salt and pepper
- ½ teaspoon of turmeric
- 1 15 ounces of can diced tomatoes with their juices
- 1 teaspoon of ground cumin
- 3 cups low-sodium vegetable broth

Directions

1. In a small bowl, add coriander, Aleppo pepper, cumin, and turmeric. Mix, set aside.

2. In a large heavy pot, heat 2 tablespoon of extra virgin olive oil over medium heat until shimmering.

3. Add onions and garlic let cook for 3 minutes, stirring occasionally.

4. Add carrots together with sweet potatoes.

5. Season with kosher salt, black pepper, and the spice mixture.

6. Increase the heat to high, let cook for 5 minutes, stirring occasionally.

7. Add diced tomatoes and broth, boil for 10 minutes.

8. Lower the heat, cover halfway and let simmer 25 minutes.

9. Stir in the baby spinach and fresh parsley.

10. Remove from heat, drizzle with extra virgin olive oil.

11. Serve and enjoy with crusty bread.

Eggplant recipe

These eggplants are perfected to velvet tender wit chickpeas and tomatoes. It is richly vegan with great garlic and onion flavors.

Ingredients

- 1 teaspoon of dry oregano
- 1.5 lb. eggplant, cut into cubes
- ½ teaspoon of organic ground turmeric
- 1 28-ounces of can chopped tomato
- ¾ teaspoon of ground cinnamon
- Fresh herbs
- Kosher salt
- Extra virgin olive oil
- 1 large yellow onion, chopped
- ½ teaspoon of black pepper
- 1 teaspoon of organic ground coriander
- 1 green bell pepper, stem and innards removed, diced
- 2 15-ounces of cans chickpeas
- 1 carrot, chopped
- 6 large garlic cloves, minced
- 2 dry bay leaves
- 1 ½ teaspoons of sweet paprika

Directions

1. Heat your oven to 400°F.
2. Place eggplant cubes in a colander over a large bowl and sprinkle with salt.
3. Set aside for 20 minutes to sweat out any bitterness.
4. Rinse with water and pat dry.
5. In a large saucepan, heat extra virgin olive oil over medium-high until shimmering without smoke.
6. Add onions together with the peppers, and chopped carrot.
7. Let cook for 3 minutes, stirring regularly.
8. Add garlic together with the bay leaf, spices, and a dash of salt.
9. Continue to cook 1 minute, stirring until fragrant.
10. Add eggplant with the chickpeas, chopped tomato, and reserved chickpea liquid. Stir.
11. Bring to a rolling boil for 10 minutes, stir often.
12. Remove from stove top, cover and transfer to oven.
13. Cook in oven for 45 minutes.
14. Add a generous drizzle of extra virgin olive oil when the eggplants are ready, then garnish with fresh herbs.
15. Serve and enjoy when warm.

Easy vegetarian pasta Faggioli recipe

This is a heaty and rusty Italian bowl with a Mediterranean twist especially roasted tomatoes, beans and some tender nutritious veggies.

Ingredients

- Extra virgin olive oil
- 6 cups of vegetable broth
- Grated Parmesan cheese
- 1 28-ounces of can fire roasted diced tomatoes
- 2 carrots, chopped
- Crushed red pepper
- 2 garlic cloves, chopped
- 1 dried bay leaf
- 1 teaspoon of dried oregano
- 1 yellow onion, chopped
- 8 ounces of small pasta
- 1 15-ounces of can cannellini beans
- 1 15-ounces of can kidney beans, rinsed and drained
- 2 celery stalks, chopped
- Salt and pepper

- ½ cup of fresh basil leaves, cut into ribbons

Directions

1. In a large boiling pot of water, cook the pasta as per the manufacturers package Directions.
2. Drain any excess water, and set aside.
3. In a large cast iron pot, heat 2 tablespoon of olive oil.
4. Sauté the onions, celery and carrots on medium-high heat for 4 minutes.
5. Add the chopped garlic with the bay leaf and dried oregano.
6. Cook for more 2 minutes, stirring occasionally.
7. Add the roasted diced tomatoes with the vegetable broth, cannellini beans, and kidney beans.
8. Season with salt and pepper.
9. Boil, then reduce the heat to simmer.
10. Cover the pot with a lid with a small opening. Simmer for 15 minutes.
11. Bring to a medium-high heat.
12. Stir in the pasta until warmed through.
13. Stir in the fresh basil, and remove from heat.
14. Transfer to serving bowls and top with crushed red pepper.
15. Serve and enjoy with crusty bread.

Cinnamon roasted sweet potatoes

These potatoes are best roasted with red onions. The hint of cinnamon gives this recipe a deeper depth of flavor.

Ingredients

- 2 small red onions cut into large pieces
- 3 lb. sweet potatoes peeled and cut into cubes
- Black pepper
- 1 teaspoon of ground cinnamon
- Kosher salt
- Extra virgin olive oil
- ¾ teaspoon of ground allspice

Directions

1. Begin by preheating your oven to 400°F.
2. Place the sweet potato cubes together with the onion pieces in a large mixing bowl.
3. Add a drizzle of extra virgin olive oil.
4. Add salt, pepper, cinnamon and allspice. Toss.
5. Shift to a sheet pan.

6. Spread the sweet potatoes and onions well in one single layer without overcrowding.

7. Roast for 45 minutes, tossing occasionally.

8. Serve and enjoy when the potatoes are cooked through.

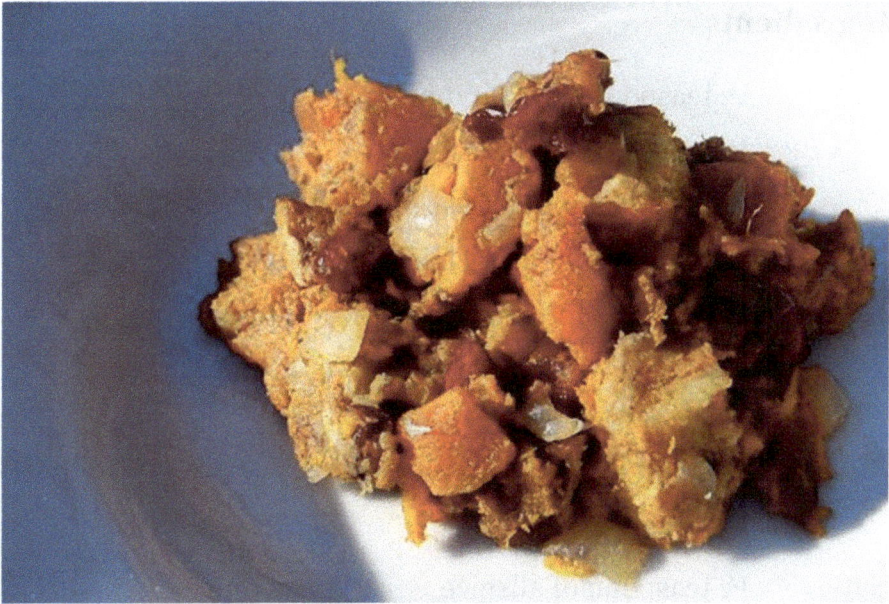

Greek stuffed tomatoes

Garlic, onions, cumin, oregano, nutmeg, and fresh herbs give this recipe thumbs up. They are baked to a perfection as they are stuffed with tomatoes.

Ingredients

- ½ teaspoon of ground nutmeg
- ½ cup of long grain rice
- ½ cup of chopped fresh spearmint
- 2 cups of canned crushed tomatoes
- 1 large red onion halved, mince ½ of the onion
- 4 garlic cloves, minced
- ½ lb. of lean ground beef
- Kosher salt and black pepper
- 6 large tomatoes
- ½ teaspoon of allspice
- ½ cup of white wine
- Extra virgin olive oil
- ¾ teaspoon of dried oregano
- ¼ cup of water
- 1 cup of chopped fresh parsley
- 1 teaspoon of ground cumin

Directions

1. Preheat your oven ready to 375°F.
2. Place olive oil in a large skillet over medium-high heat let shimmer without smoke.
3. Add chopped onions and garlic, toss.
4. Add the ground meat, season with salt, pepper, cumin, oregano, allspice, and nutmeg. Let cook for 5 minutes.
5. Add drained rice when the meat is ready.
6. Add crushed tomatoes, white wine, and water.
7. Bring the saucy mixture to a boil, turn the heat down, let simmer for 10 minutes.
8. Stir in the fresh herbs. Season with kosher salt.
9. Oil the bottom of a baking pan with extra virgin olive oil.
10. Spread chopped tomato flesh and sliced onion at the bottom of the baking dish.
11. Add the chopped tomato flesh and sliced onion to make a bed for the stuffed tomatoes.
12. Spoon the saucy meat and rice mixture into the empty tomato shells.
13. Cover the stuffed tomatoes with the reserved tops.
14. From one of the corners of your baking dish, carefully pour about ¾ cup of water.
15. Add a little pinch of salt and a generous drizzle of extra virgin olive oil on top.
16. Cover the baking dish with foil and bake in heated oven for 45 minutes.

17. Uncover let cook for more 1 hour.

18. When ready, serve and enjoy.

Carpers chicken

Although Mediterranean Sea diet focuses on fruits and vegetables, this carpers chicken is accompanied by rich vegetables.

Ingredients

- 1 lb. of boneless skinless chicken breasts
- 8 Fresh basil leaves
- Balsamic glaze or balsamic reduction
- Black pepper
- Extra virgin olive oil
- Kosher salt
- 4 slices low-sodium fresh mozzarella cheese
- Basil pesto
- 4 thick slices of ripe tomatoes

Directions

1. Pat chicken dry and season with salt and pepper.
2. Heat an indoor griddle then, drizzle with bit of extra virgin olive oil to coat bottom of pan.
3. Place in the chicken let cook for 5 minutes on each side.

4. At the last couple minutes of cooking, top each piece of chicken with a bit of the basil pesto, then add mozzarella slice on top.

5. Remove from heat source.

6. Add fresh basil leaves and tomato slices on top.

7. Sprinkle with fresh basil ribbons.

8. Serve and enjoy.

Mediterranean potato hash with asparagus, chickpeas and poached eggs

This is a colorful Mediterranean breakfast topped with chickpeas and poached eggs.

Ingredients

- ½ cup of crumbled feta
- 2 garlic cloves, chopped
- 2 russet potatoes, diced
- Salt and pepper
- 1 cup of chopped fresh parsley,
- 1 cup of canned chickpeas, drained and rinsed
- 1 small red onion, finely chopped
- 1 teaspoon of coriander
- 1 lb.. baby asparagus, hard ends removed, chopped into ¼ inch pieces
- Extra virgin olive oil
- 1 ½ tsp ground allspice
- 1 teaspoon of Za'atar
- 2 Roma tomatoes, chopped
- 1 teaspoon of dried oregano
- 1 small yellow onion, chopped

- Pinch sugar
- 4 eggs
- 1 teaspoon of sweet paprika
- Water
- 1 teaspoon of White Vinegar

Directions

1. Heat olive oil in a large cast-iron skillet.
2. Add the chopped onions, garlic and potatoes with the heat turned low.
3. Season with salt and pepper let cook for 7 minutes, stirring frequently until the potatoes are tender.
4. Add the chickpeas together with asparagus, a dash more salt and pepper and the spices. Stir to combine.
5. Continue to cook for 7 minutes.
6. Lower heat to keep the potato hash warm, stir regularly.
7. Boil water to a steady simmer then add 1 teaspoon of vinegar.
8. Break the eggs into a bowl.
9. Stir the simmering water gently and carefully slide the eggs in let cook for 3 minutes.
10. Season with salt and pepper.
11. Remove the potato hash from the heat and add the chopped red onions, tomatoes, feta and parsley.
12. Top with the poached eggs.
13. Serve and enjoy.

Fried eggplant recipe with green peppers and tomatoes

Vegan, vegetarian alike, this recipe is a perfect option for vegans and vegetarians in love with awesome Mediterranean Sea diet.

Ingredients

- 2 large green bell peppers washed, dried, sliced
- 5 garlic cloves Roughly chopped
- 2 teaspoon of sumac
- ½ cup of fresh mint
- 2 teaspoon of white vinegar
- 6 large slicing tomato washed, dried, sliced in rounds
- ½ cup of healthy cooking oil
- 1 large eggplant washed, dried, sliced in rounds
- kosher salt
- ¼ cup of walnut hearts

Directions

1. Spread eggplant slices on paper towels and sprinkle generously with kosher salt.
2. Let sit for 30 minutes to sweat out any bitterness. Pat dry.

3. Heat oil on medium-high heat let shimmer without smoke.

4. Fry the green peppers, skin side down, until tender.

5. Drain any excess oil, then sprinkle with a little salt and sumac.

6. In the same frying pan, fry the eggplant flip over to balance the fry.

7. Sprinkle with sumac.

8. Then, fry the tomatoes for 2 minutes, add the garlic, let cook for 5 minutes, tossing gently.

9. Lower the heat to add 2 tablespoons of vinegar, salt, and pinch of sumac.

10. Turn heat off when tomatoes are releasing juices and turning bright orange.

11. Layer a bit of the eggplant at the bottom, then add green peppers, then the saucy tomatoes on top.

12. Repeat this step until the veggies are all on the platter.

13. Garnish with fresh mint and walnut hearts.

14. Serve and enjoy with Lebanese rice.

Crunchy roasted chickpeas

This is a quickie Mediterranean diet snack. It requires few ingredients especially salt and olive oil for the roast.

Ingredients

- Kosher salt
- 2 15 ounces cans of chickpeas, drained and rinsed
- Extra virgin olive oil
- Seasoning of your choice

Directions

1. Drain and pat dry chickpeas.
2. Heat your oven to 400°F.
3. Spread the chickpeas well on a bare baking sheet.
4. Drizzle with extra virgin olive oil and season with kosher salt. Toss.
5. Roast in heated oven for 35 minutes, shaking the pan every 10 minutes.
6. When chickpeas turn a deeper golden brown and the exterior is nice and crispy, they are ready.
7. Season roasted chickpeas.
8. Serve and enjoy.

Mediterranean style okra recipe

So far, this is the most amazing recipe among the Mediterranean Sea diet. Combining okra with onions and garlic with hot peppers, lime juice is remarkably perfect for a Mediterranean meal.

Ingredients

- Juice of ½ lime
- 1 small onion chopped
- 1 tomato sliced into rounds
- 4 garlic cloves minced
- ½ cup of water
- 1 lb.. frozen or fresh cut of okra sliced into rounds
- Salt and pepper
- 1 teaspoon of ground allspice
- ½ teaspoon of coriander
- 2 small green chills
- ½ teaspoon of paprika
- Extra virgin olive oil
- 1 ½ cup of crushed tomatoes

Directions

1. Begin by heating olive oil in a large skillet over medium-high until shimmering without smoke.
2. Lower the heat, add the onions together with the garlic and chopped jalapeno peppers.
3. Let cook for 5 minutes stir frequently.
4. Add the okra and sauté for 7 minutes over medium-high heat.
5. Season with kosher salt, black pepper and spices. Toss.
6. Add the crushed tomatoes and water. Stir to combine.
7. Add the tomato slices on top and boil.
8. Lower the heat, cover most of the way let okra simmer for 20 – 25 minutes.
9. Uncover and add juice of ½ lime accordingly.
10. Remove from heat and serve over rice .
11. Enjoy.

Mediterranean salmon and vegetable quinoa

This Mediterranean salmon vegetable recipe cannot be underestimated in regards to its protein content. It is fully packed with healthy protein from vegetables and roasted spices with salmon fillets.

Ingredients

- ¾ cup of English cucumbers, diced, seeded
- ½ teaspoon of kosher salt
- ¼ cup of red onion, finely diced
- zest of one lemon
- ½ teaspoon of kosher salt
- 1 cup of quinoa, uncooked
- ¼ teaspoon of black pepper
- 8 lemon wedges
- 1 teaspoon of cumin
- 4 basil leaves, thinly sliced
- 1 cup of cherry tomatoes, sliced in half
- ½ teaspoon of paprika
- 20 ounces of salmon fillets
- ¼ cup of parsley, chopped fresh

Directions

1. Boil I cup of quinoa, water and salt in a medium saucepan.
2. Cook at reduced heat for 20 minutes as instructed on the package till fluffy.
3. Turn off the heat allow it to settle for 5 minutes covered.
4. Mix in the tomatoes, cucumbers, basil, onions, and lemon zest.
5. In another separate small bowl, combine cumin, salt, pepper, and paprika.
6. Line a sheet pan with a foil, grease with olive oil.
7. Move the salmon fillets to the pan. Make sure to coat evenly on each surface with spice mixture.
8. Place the lemon wedges at the edges of the pan.
9. Broil on high heat for 8 – 10 minutes with the rack placed in the lower third of the oven till salmon is ready.
10. Sprinkle with parsley.
11. Serve and enjoy with roasted lemon wedges and vegetable quinoa.

Vegan tofu tikka masala

Tons of rich flavors feature in this Mediterranean vegan dish. This recipe using sesame oil and coconut milk in the place of butter making it a healthier option for your meal.

Ingredients

- ½ large head of cauliflower
- 1 ¼ teaspoon of Sea Salt
- Salt and pepper to taste
- ½ cup of red onion finely diced
- ½ cup full fat coconut milk
- ¼ cup of fresh ginger finely grated
- 1 ½ teaspoon of paprika
- 12 ounces extra firm tofu
- 1/8 teaspoon of nutmeg
- ¼ teaspoon of cayenne pepper
- 1 ½ teaspoon of ground cumin
- 4 cloves garlic minced
- 2 14 ounce cans of diced tomatoes
- ½ teaspoon of turmeric
- cilantro to garnish
- 3 teaspoon of sesame oil

Directions

1. Begin by preparing your tofu by draining excess liquid.
2. Wrap well within paper towels with a heavy material put on it for at least 10 minutes.
3. In a skillet over medium temperature, add sesame oil followed by cubed tofu pieces.
4. Season briefly with sea salt and pepper flip to let brown.
5. Remove from pan.
6. Add chopped garlic, onions, and grated ginger in the sesame oil balance.
7. Sauté for 5 minutes until onions are translucent.
8. Add all spices to the pan, including onion and ginger mixture.
9. Pulse diced tomatoes in a blender, process until somewhat smooth.
10. Transfer tomatoes into the pan, stir to combine.
11. Add the tofu in, simmer for 10 minutes over low heat.
12. Then add coconut milk, warm on low boil.
13. Season with cayenne and sea salt.
14. Place cauliflower in a food processor bowl.
15. Process until broken into pieces.
16. Add sesame oil and cauliflower over high heat.
17. Sauté briefly for 3 minutes.
18. Season with sea salt and pepper.
19. Serve tofu tikka masala over cauliflower and enjoy with cilantro.

Mediterranean couscous

This couscous recipe is typically with nutritious flavors from herbs, zippy lemon, variety of veggies. As such, this is a versatile recipe for breakfast, lunch and dinner.

Ingredients

- ⅓ cup of extra virgin olive oil
- 2 garlic cloves, minced
- ½ English cucumber, finely chopped
- Salt and pepper
- Private Reserve extra virgin olive oil
- Water
- 2 cups of grape tomatoes, halved
- 3 oz. fresh baby mozzarella
- 15 oz. can of chickpeas, drained and rinsed
- 14 oz. can of artichoke hearts
- 1 teaspoon of dill weed
- ⅓ cup of finely chopped red onions
- 1 large lemon juice
- 2 cups of Pearl Couscous
- ½ cup of pitted Kalamata olives
- 15-20 fresh basil leaves, roughly chopped

Directions

1. Put vinaigrette ingredients in a bowl. Whisk all to combine.
2. In a medium-sized pot, heat 2 tablespoons of olive oil .
3. Let couscous Sauté in the olive oil shortly to turn golden brown.
4. Next, add 3 cups of boiling water continue to cook as per package instruction.
5. Drain and keep for later.
6. In a separate large mixing dish, combine all ingredients except basil and mozzarella.
7. Add couscous with the basil mix.
8. Whisk the lemon-dill vinaigrette. Add to couscous salad.
9. Mix to combine.
10. Test and season accordingly.
11. Blend in the mozzarella cheese and finally garnish with basil.
12. Serve and enjoy.

Stuffed peppers

The recipe derives its taste from rich meat packed with flavors and herbs as well as chickpeas. It a gluten free vegetarian dish for dinner and lunch or breakfast.

Ingredients

- 1 can of cannellini beans, drained and rinsed
- 4 cloves garlic, minced
- ½ cup of Feta cheese
- 5 cups of low-sodium vegetable broth
- 1 can of diced tomatoes
- 1 cup of carrots diced
- 1 cup of faro, rinsed
- 1 tablespoons of fresh lemon juice
- 1 cup of chopped celery
- 1 teaspoon of dried oregano
- 1 bay leaf
- 1 cup of chopped yellow onion
- Salt
- 2 tablespoon of olive oil
- ½ cup of packed parsley sprigs
- 4 cups of packed chopped kale

Directions

1. Begin by heating oil over medium-high heat in a large pot.
2. Next, add carrots, onion and celery, let Sauté for 3 minutes.
3. Add garlic Sauté briefly.
4. Stir in faro, vegetable broth, oregano, tomatoes, bay leaf, season with salt accordingly.
5. Add parsley to the soup, let boil over low heat.
6. Cover let simmer for 19 – 21 minutes.
7. Remove parsley to stir in kale and kale, let cook for 13 – 15 minutes.
8. Add cannellini beans, heat for 1 minute.
9. Discard bay leaf and stir in lemon juice with extra vegetable broth.
10. Serve warm and enjoy topped with feta cheese.

Easy Falafel meal

Ingredients

- Lemon
- ¼ teaspoon of Garlic Powder
- pinch each salt & pepper
- ½ cup of white onion
- ¼ cup of oat flour
- 2 tablespoons of tahini
- 3-4 tablespoons of avocado oil
- 4 cup of lettuce
- 2 tomatoes diced
- 1.5 teaspoon cumin
- 1/3 cup of chopped fresh parsley
- 1 Cucumber diced
- 1-15 ounce can chickpeas drained and rinsed
- 1 red onion sliced thin

Directions

1. Add chickpeas, parsley, garlic powder, onions, tahini, cumin, and pepper to a blender, pulse to combined.
2. Add oat flour pulse again.
3. Then over high temperature, heat a large skillet with avocado oil.

4. Scoop out falafel mixture, form into patties.

5. Add falafel patties after the pan has heat up, let cook for 5 minutes.

6. Repeat for all falafel patties until they turn golden brown.

7. Divide lettuce, cucumber, tomato, and red onion in 4 dishes.

8. Add falafel on top.

9. Serve and enjoy with tahini or lemon.

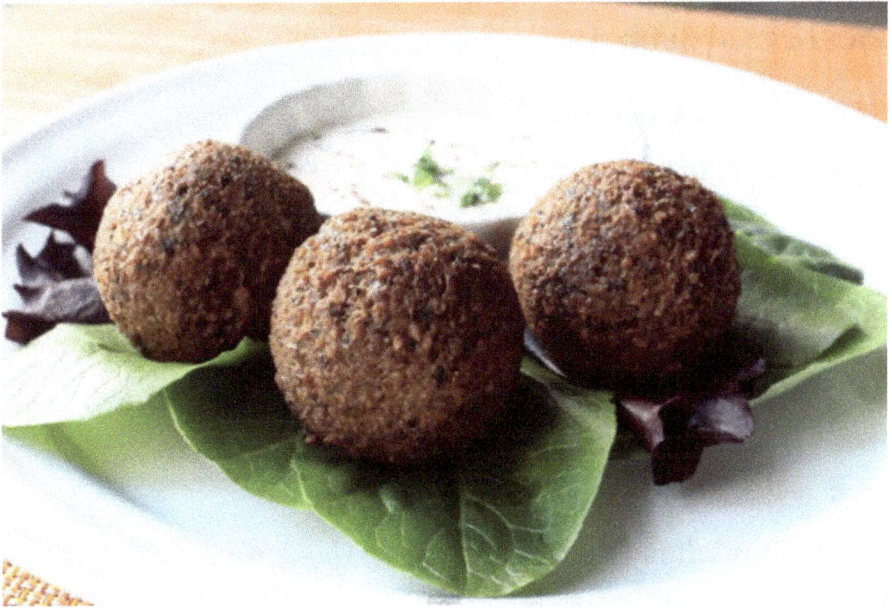

Pan seared salmon

To sear salmon, you need warm variety of spices which can be topped with a salsa fresca a Mediterranean style. Furthermore, the other ingredients used to make this recipe are quite simple especially garlic, pepper, cumin and coriander.

Ingredients

Pan Seared Salmon

- 1 teaspoon paprika
- ½ teaspoon ground cumin
- 1 teaspoon grated lemon zest
- ½ teaspoon ground coriander
- ¼ teaspoon salt
- ½ teaspoon granulated onion
- ¼ teaspoon black pepper
- Olive or avocado oil
- 4 salmon fillets skinned
- Pinch cayenne pepper
- 1 teaspoon granulated garlic

Mediterranean Salsa Fresca

- ¼ yellow bell pepper, finely diced
- 2 tablespoons finely diced red onion

- Black pepper
- 1 teaspoon chopped fresh dill
- 1 teaspoon chopped flat-leaf parsley
- Salt
- 2 tablespoons pitted Kalamata olives, diced
- 1 cup small cherry or sugar tomatoes, quartered
- ½ teaspoon grated lemon zest
- 1 small Persian cucumber, finely diced
- 1 teaspoon lemon juice

Toasted Couscous

- 1 tablespoon olive oil
- 1 cup couscous
- 1 tablespoon chopped parsley
- 1 clove garlic, pressed through garlic press
- 1 ¼ cup water
- Couple pinches of salt

Directions

1. Firstly, Place the salmon fillets onto in a large bowl
2. Drizzle 2 tablespoon of oil, sprinkle with paprika, cumin, garlic, onion, salt, coriander, pepper, cayenne and lemon zest, and toss.
3. Let marinate for not less than 1 hour.

4. As you wait for the salmon, combine all ingredients mix to combine. Ensure to keep refrigerated when covered.

5. Again put another medium saucepan to heat over medium temperature.

6. Add in the couscous and toast for 1 minute. Remove and keep for later.

7. In the same pan, add water with salt, olive oil, and garlic. Stir to combine.

8. Simmer thoroughly.

9. Pour in couscous, stir.

10. Turn off heat, leave covered for 4 – 7 minutes to soften.

11. Add the chopped parsley, make sure it stays warm.

12. Put a large skillet to heat spread with oil.

13. Add in salmon fillets, let them sear on every side for 4 – 5 minutes. Repeat step for the other side.

14. Top seared salmon with Mediterranean Salsa Fresca.

15. Serve and enjoy.

Candied oranges dipped in chocolate

This recipe is for a sweet tasty treat for a perfect holiday to enjoy Mediterranean Sea diet. The chocolates can be substituted with cupcakes if you like.

Ingredients

- 3.5 ounces of Dark Chocolate
- 1 Large Orange, organic
- Coarse Salt
- 1 cup of Granulated Sugar
- 1 cup of Water

Directions

1. Cut the oranges into thin slices.
2. Heat water and sugar in a large pot until the sugar has dissolved.
3. Add the orange slices in a manner that they are spread around without covering each other totally.
4. Let simmer for 40 minutes on a low heat. Turn occasionally.

5. Transfer slices onto a wire rack when ready, let them cool completely.

6. It is fine to cool on a fridge to speed up the cooling process.

7. Melt the chocolate over a pot of simmering water.

8. Dip half of each slice in chocolate.

9. Place the dipped one's onto a tray lined with a sheet of aluminum foil.

10. Sprinkle with salt.

11. Shift all of them into the fridge.

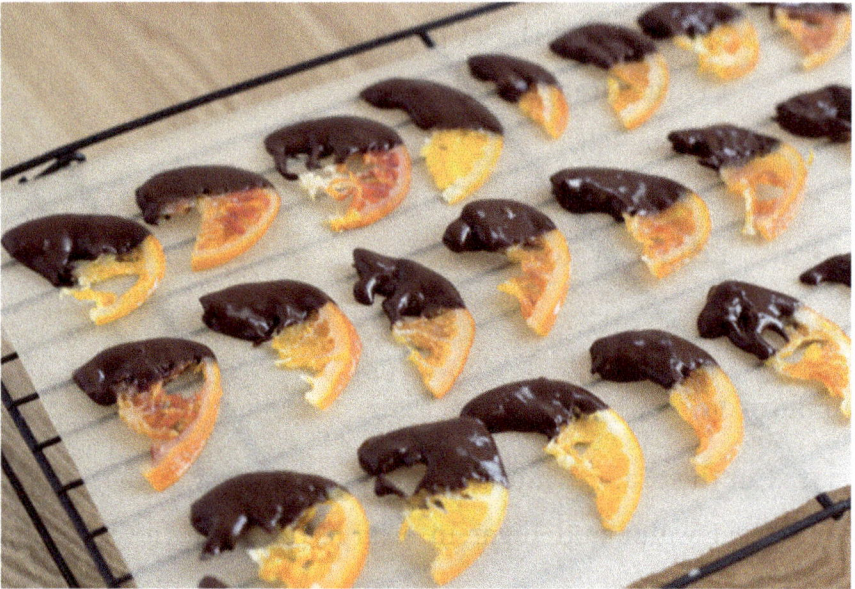

12. Serve an enjoy.

Walnut crescent cookies

If you want taste and know divine taste covered in a powdered sugar, look no further, walnut crescent cookies can give you that same exact taste.

Ingredients

- 2 tablespoons of vanilla sugar
- 11/4 cup of all-purpose flour
- ½ cup of powdered sugar
- 1 stick unsalted butter
- ⅔ cup of ground walnuts
- 4 tablespoons of powdered sugar
- 1 teaspoon of vanilla essence

Directions

1. In a large mixing bowl, begin by combining sifted powdered sugar, sifted flour, and ground walnuts.
2. Next, add vanilla essence and mix thoroughly.
3. Then, grate chilled butter.
4. Add to the bowl.
5. Combine all the ingredients using your bare hands until dough is formed in 3 minutes or so.

6. Place into a Ziploc bag allow it to chill for 30 minutes in the fridge.
7. As it refrigerates, get a small bowl and place extra powdered sugar with vanilla sugar in it and keep aside.
8. Take a piece of the dough and roll into a ball then into a sausage.
9. Shape the sausage into a crescent.
10. Place onto a baking tray with baking parchment.
11. For the remaining dough, repeat this step.
12. Bake in a ready heated oven at 400°F for 8 minutes or so.
13. Allow it to cool down completely on the tray when already fried.
14. Transfer to a plat and dip with powdered sugar to coat.
15. Serve and enjoy.

Caramel apple dip

The caramel apple dip is a perfect and excellent choice for family gatherings with only 3 ingredients, it is a quickie in only 2 minutes with absolutely no cooking and frying needed.

Ingredients

- Caramels
- ½ cup of Dulce de leche
- 2 – 3 apples, cut into small pieces
- ½ cup of cream cheese

Directions

1. In a bowl, mix the cream cheese together with the Dulce de leech until smooth.
2. Cut the apples into quarters after rinsing.
3. Remove the hard parts.
4. Further cut every quarter into 6 slices
5. Serve and enjoy.

Easy lemon cupcakes

Lemon is a nutritious fruit fantastic for a Mediterranean Sea diet. The lemon gives this recipe a flavorful taste super moist topped with vanilla mascarpone cream cheese frosting.

Ingredients

- ½ cup of granulated sugar

- 3/4 cup of all-purpose flour

  - 2 eggs, at room temperature
  - 2 teaspoon of baking powder
  - 1/4 teaspoon of vanilla essence
  - 3 small lemons, juice only
  - A pinch of salt
  - ½ cup of powdered sugar
  - 1 tablespoon of lemon juice
  - 1 stick unsalted butter , softened
  - 9 ounces of mascarpone cheese
  - ½ cup of cream cheese

Directions

1. Firstly, begin by preheating your oven to 360°F.

2. Juice all the lemons without the seeds, keep for later.
3. In a mixing dish, beat the butter together with sugar until creamy in 3 minutes.
4. Add the eggs and mix well.
5. Combine the flour together with the baking powder and salt.
6. Add this to the cupcake batter and mix until smooth.
7. Pour in the lemon juice and mix thoroughly for the last time.
8. Place the paper cases in a muffin tray.
9. Using a pipe, pipe the batter into paper cases.
10. Let bake for 15 minutes.
11. If you the inserted skewer comes out clean, it is an indication that the cupcakes are ready.
12. Remove from the oven.
13. Pour in the balance of the lemon juice over each cupcake (2 spoons per cake).
14. Allow it to cool down completely.
15. Shift all the ingredients into a mixing bowl.
16. Combine them using an electric mixer until smooth.
17. Serve and enjoy.

Lemon blueberry poke cake from scratch

This is a typical moist sponge soft recipe featuring blueberry sauce and creamy ricotta with a hint of lemon to give it the attractive flavor for a Mediterranean Sea diet.

Ingredients

- ½ cup of powdered sugar
- 1½ teaspoon of baking powder
- 1 cup of fresh blueberries
- ½ lemon, juice only
- 1/4 cup of sunflower oil
- 1/4 cup of water
- 1 cup of all-purpose flour
- 3 medium eggs, yolks and whites separated
- ½ cup of granulated sugar
- 2 cups of frozen blueberries
- Lemon zest
- 3/4 cup of granulated sugar
- ½ lemon, juice only
- 8 ounce of mascarpone
- 1/4 cup water
- 8 ounce of ricotta

Directions

1. Start by beating the egg whites until soft peaks forms, keep for later.
2. In another separate mixing dish, whisk the egg yolks together with sugar until creamy.
3. Sift in flour mixed with baking powder. Mix properly.
4. Add oil together with water, continue to mix with an electric mixer until smooth.
5. Fold in the egg whites and pour the batter in a rectangular baking dish.
6. Begin baking for 15 minutes at 375°F.
7. Allow it to cool down.
8. Pierce in holes when completely cooled.
9. As the cake is in the oven, heat up the blueberries together with the water, sugar, and lemon juice in a sauce pan.
10. Over low heat simmer for 7 minutes.
11. Turn off heat, keep aside.
12. In another separate bowl, combine ricotta together with the freshly squeezed lemon juice, mascarpone, and sugar.
13. Place in the electric mixer mix until well combined.
14. Pour the blueberries and their juice over the cake sponge.
15. Then, spread the ricotta layer over.
16. Refrigerate to chill.
17. Serve and enjoy with blueberries and or grated lemon zest if you like.

Chocolate mango cheesecake parfait

This is an excellent choice for passing through the summer season. It combines Oreo cookies with fresh mangoes, mango cheesecake and chocolate for a tastier breakfast for a Mediterranean diet.

Ingredients

- 3 tablespoons of lemon juice
- 1 fresh mango
- 12 ounces of cream cheese
- 1 packet of oreo cookies
- ½ cup of whipping cream
- 2 tablespoons of unsweetened cocoa powder
- ½ cup of powdered sugar

Instruction

1. Begin by cutting the mango, scoop the flesh from one half out.
2. Puree in a food processor, keep aside.
3. The remaining half should be cut into slices.

4. Whip the cream until soft peaks form in a small mixing dish.
5. Add the cream cheese together with the powdered sugar and mix to combined.
6. Divide this mixture equally between 2 dishes.
7. Add pureed mango and lemon juice in one.
8. Fill the next one with cocoa powder.
9. Mix both until well combined.
10. You can start with a whole Oreo cookie.
11. Then a mango cheesecake layer, fresh mango slices.
12. Then, lastly, place the chocolate cheesecake layer.
13. Repeat this until everything is finished.
14. Garnish with some Oreo crumb.
15. Refrigerate for 1 hour to chill.
16. Serve and enjoy.

Raspberry mint ice pops

Mint is one element in this recipe that gives it a refreshing taste and keeping you hooked onto it. The raspberry flavor can be felt through the entire raspberry.

Ingredients

- 1½ cup of Fresh Raspberries
- 1 Wedge of Lemon
- ⅓ cup of Honey
- 10 Mint Leaves
- 1 cup of Water

Directions

1. In a small sauce pan, combine the honey, water, together with 5 mint leaves.
2. Heat this up without boiling until the honey is melted. Keep for later.
3. Then, puree the raspberries including the remaining mint leaves in a food processor.
4. Sieve the mixture to remove any seeds in it.
5. Make sure to remove any mint leaves from honey water at this stage.

6. Add in the pureed raspberries.

7. Squeeze in the lemon mix thoroughly.

8. Then pour it into popsicle molds.

9. Freeze for at least 8 hours, otherwise 12 hours is best.

10. Serve and enjoy.

Baked lemon garlic salmon

This is an amazing recipe. The garlic fills it with its aromatic flavor.

Ingredients

- 2 teaspoons of dry oregano
- Kosher salt
- ½ teaspoon of black pepper
- ½ lemon, sliced into rounds
- 1 teaspoon of sweet paprika
- Parsley for garnish
- Zest of 1 large lemon
- 2 lb. salmon fillet
- Juice of 2 lemons
- 5 garlic cloves, chopped
- Extra virgin olive oil

Directions

1. Heat your oven to 375°F.
2. In a small mixing dish, mix together the lemon juice with garlic, lemon zest, extra virgin olive oil, paprika, oregano, and black pepper. Whisk well.

3. Organize a sheet pan. Make sure it is lined with a large piece of foil with the top brushed with extra virgin olive oil.

4. Next, pat the salmon dry, let season on both sides with kosher salt.

5. Place it on the foiled sheet pan.

6. Top with lemon garlic sauce evenly.

7. Fold foil over the salmon.

8. Then, proceed to bake for 20 minutes. The salmon should be almost cooked through on the side that is thicker.

9. Remove out and open foil to uncover the top of the salmon.

10. Place under the broiler briefly.

11. Serve and enjoy.

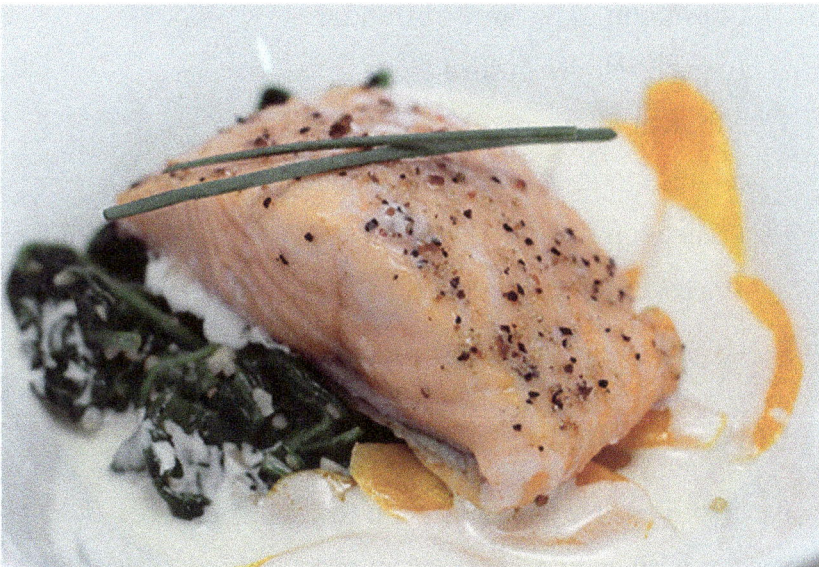

Baked fish with garlic and basil

The fish comes out tender infused with aromatic garlic flavor and the basil. It also blends in some citrus and extra virgin olive oil for a better Mediterranean diet.

Ingredients

- 2 bell peppers any color, sliced
- 15 basil leaves, sliced into ribbons
- Salt and pepper
- 1 ½ tsp dry oregano
- 2 shallots, peeled and sliced
- 1 teaspoon of ground coriander
- 10 garlic cloves, minced
- 2 lb. fish fillet
- 6 tablespoon of extra virgin olive oil
- 1 teaspoon of sweet paprika
- Juice of 1 lemon

Directions

1. Pat fish fillet dry with a kitchen towel.
2. Season with salt and pepper on every side.
3. Place the fish in a large zip-top bag.

4. Then, add the oregano, paprika, coriander, basil, minced garlic, extra virgin olive oil and lemon juice in to the bag, massage to evenly coat the fish.
5. Place in the fridge to marinated for 1 hour.
6. Heat your oven to 425°F.
7. Organize the bell peppers and shallots in the bottom of a baking dish.
8. Place the fish on top and pour the marinade over.
9. Bake in heated oven for 15 minutes.
10. Let cool briefly.
11. Serve and enjoy.

Green shakshuka recipe

This recipe is Mediterranean but takes a new classic turn with power greens especially spinach, Brussel sprouts and herbs mainly kale.

Ingredients

- Crumbled feta
- ¼ cup of extra virgin olive oil
- 1 green onion, trimmed
- 1 teaspoon of coriander
- 8 ounces of Brussels sprouts
- ½ large red onion, finely chopped
- Handful fresh parsley
- 1 teaspoon of Aleppo pepper
- 3 garlic cloves, minced
- 1 large bunch kale
- 2 cups of baby spinach
- ¾ teaspoon of cumin
- 4 large eggs
- Kosher salt
- Juice of ½ lemon

Directions

1. In a skillet that has a lid, heat the extra virgin olive oil until shimmering without smoke over medium heat.
2. Add the sliced Brussels sprouts, sprinkle with a dash of kosher salt.
3. Let cook for 6 minutes, keep tossing occasionally to soften uniformly.
4. Lower the heat.
5. Add the onions and garlic together, continue to cook for 4 more minutes, tossing regularly.
6. Add the kale, let wilt in 5 minutes as you toss.
7. Add the spinach and toss to combine.
8. Season with a pinch of kosher salt and adjust accordingly.
9. Add all the spices and toss to combine.
10. Then, add ½ cup of water.
11. Regulate the heat to medium continue to cook for 10 minutes when covered. Make sure at this point the kale is wilted totally.
12. Stir in the lemon juice.
13. Make 4 wells using your spoon.
14. Crack an egg into each well.
15. Do not forget to season each egg with some of salt. Cook for 4 minutes with the pan covered.
16. Remove from the heat.
17. Add more drizzle of extra virgin olive oil. Optional.

18. Garnish with the parsley, fresh green onions, and feta if you desire.
19. Serve and enjoy with bread or pita immediately.

Mediterranean backed cod

Unlike other recipes, the Mediterranean backed cod utilizes fewer spices mainly lemon juice, massive amount of garlic and olive oil in 15 minutes.

Ingredients

- ¾ teaspoon of salt
- ½ teaspoon of black pepper
- ¾ teaspoon of sweet Spanish paprika
- 1.5 lb. Cod fillet pieces
- ¼ cup chopped fresh parsley leaves
- 5 tablespoons of fresh lemon juice
- ¾ teaspoon of ground cumin
- 2 tablespoons of melted butter
- ⅓ cup of all-purpose flour
- 5 garlic cloves, peeled and minced
- 1 teaspoon of ground coriander
- 5 tablespoons of Private Reserve extra virgin olive oil

Directions

1. Preheat your oven ready to 400°F.

2. In a small mixing dish, mix lemon juice together with the olive oil, and melted butter. Keep for later.

3. In another separate mixing dish, mix all-purpose flour together with the spices, salt and pepper. Keep aside for later.

4. Pat fish fillet dry using a towel.

5. Dip fish in the lemon juice mixture, then dip in the flour mixture.

6. Shake off excess flour. Keep the lemon juice later.

7. In a cast iron skillet, heat 2 tablespoon of olive oil over medium temperature till shimmering without smoke.

8. Add the salmon and sear on each side. Cook briefly and remove from heat.

9. Add minced garlic to the balance of the lemon juice mixture, mix.

10. Drizzle all over the fish fillets.

11. Now you can bake in the heated oven for 10 minutes.

12. Remove from heat and sprinkle chopped parsley.

13. Serving and enjoy immediately with Lebanese rice or traditional Greek salad.

Italian oven roasted vegetables

If you are looking a massive blast of Mediterranean diet vegetables combination, then look no more. This recipe combines several vegetables that are gluten free and highly healthy.

Ingredients

- Freshly grated Parmesan cheese
- 12 ounces of baby potatoes, scrubbed
- 12 ounces of Campari tomatoes, grape
- 1 teaspoon of dried thyme
- 2 zucchini or summer squash, cut into 1-inch pieces
- 12 large garlic cloves peeled
- Extra virgin olive oil
- ½ tablespoon of dried oregano
- 8 ounces of baby Bella mushrooms cleaned, trimmed
- Salt and pepper
- Crushed red pepper flakes optional

Directions

1. Expressly, preheat your oven ready to 425°F.

2. Place the mushrooms together with the veggies and garlic in a large mixing dish.

3. Drizzle with olive oil.

4. Add the thyme, dried oregano, salt, and pepper. Toss to combine.

5. Only take the potatoes and spread them on a baking pan slightly oiled.

6. Roast for 10 minutes in the preheated oven.

7. Add the mushrooms together with the remaining vegetables after removing the potatoes from the oven.

8. Return to the oven for further 20-minute roasting or until the veggies are tender.

9. If you desire, sprinkle with of freshly grated Parmesan cheese.

10. Serve and enjoy immediately.

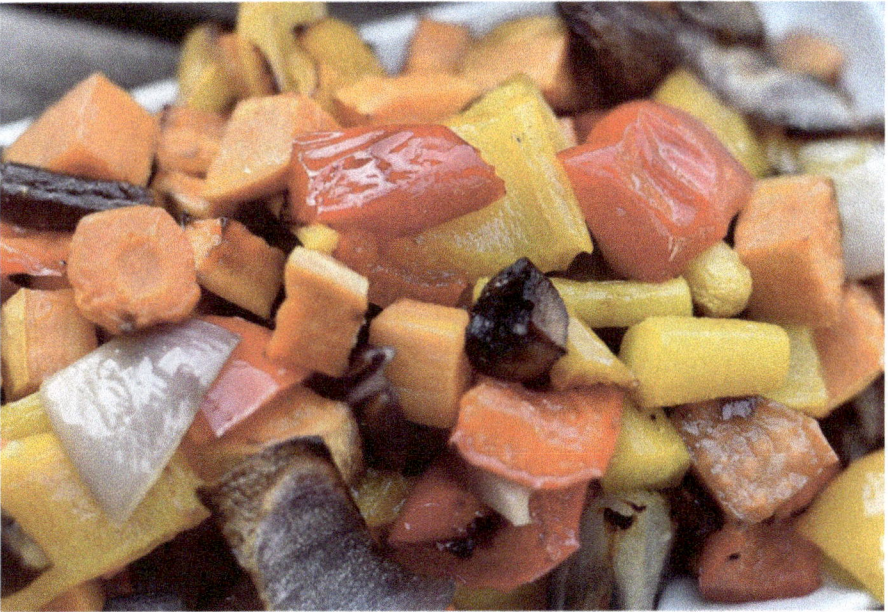

Shrimp pasta recipe Mediterranean diet style

Shrimp pasta is flavored with garlic, onions, and lemon juice. It gets ready in only 20 minutes.

Ingredients

- 1 lemon zested and juiced
- Kosher salt
- 1 lb. of large shrimp peeled and deveined
- Parmesan cheese to your liking
- ½ red onion chopped
- ¾ lb. of thin spaghetti
- 1 teaspoon of dry oregano
- 3 vine ripe tomatoes chopped
- Black pepper
- ½ teaspoon of red pepper flakes
- Extra virgin olive oil
- 1 cup of dry white wine
- 5 garlic cloves minced
- Large handful chopped fresh parsley

Directions

1. Begin by cooking the pasta in salted boiling water as per the manufacturers instruction on the package.
2. Drain any excess water and reserving some for later.
3. As the pasta is cooking, in a large pan heat extra virgin olive oil over medium temperature until it shimmers without smoke.
4. Cook the shrimp for 3 minutes on each side until pink.
5. Shift the shrimp to a side plate.
6. In the same pan, reduce the heat to medium-low.
7. Then, add the onions together with the oregano, garlic, and red pepper flakes.
8. Continue to cook for further 2 minutes, stirring constantly.
9. Add the wine to the pan, be sure to scrape up any pieces of garlic and onions.
10. Cook the wine briefly.
11. Stir in the lemon juice and lemon zest.
12. Add the chopped parsley and tomatoes, toss vigorously for 15 seconds.
13. Season with Kosher salt and adjust accordingly.
14. Now, add the cooked pasta to the pan, let toss to coat.
15. Then, add some of the reserved pasta starchy water.
16. Add the cooked shrimp.
17. Allow the shrimp to warm through briefly.

18. Remove from heat and sprinkle a little grated parmesan cheese and red pepper flakes.
19. Serve and enjoy immediately.

Moroccan vegetable tagine recipe

In this recipe, the Moroccan flavors take control of the taste with vegetables stew packed balance. The recipe is gluten free with vegetables and fruits.

Ingredients

- 10 garlic cloves, peeled and chopped
- 2 large russet potatoes, peeled and cubed
- 1 lemon, juice of
- 1 large sweet potato, peeled and cubed
- 1 teaspoon of ground cinnamon
- Handful fresh parsley leaves
- Salt
- 1 teaspoon of ground coriander
- ¼ cup of Private Reserve extra virgin olive oil
- 2 medium yellow onions, peeled and chopped
- 1 tablespoon of Harissa spice blend
- ½ teaspoon of ground turmeric
- 2 cups of canned whole peeled tomatoes
- 2 large carrots, peeled and chopped
- ½ cup of heaping chopped dried apricot

- 1 quart of low sodium vegetable broth
- 2 cups cooked chickpeas

Directions

1. Heat oil over low heat until just shimmering without smoke in a large pot.
2. Add onions and increase heat to medium.
3. Then, Sauté for 5 minutes, tossing frequently.
4. Now add the garlic and the chopped veggies.
5. Season with salt and spices. Toss again to combine.
6. Cook this combination for 7 minutes on medium-high temperature, regularly stir with a wooden spoon.
7. Add tomatoes together with the apricot and broth.
8. Season again with small dash of salt.
9. Maintain the heat on medium-high, continue to cook for 10 more minutes.
10. Then lower the heat to simmer when covered for 25 minutes or until veggies are tender.
11. Next, stir in chickpeas let cook for 5 minutes more on low heat.
12. Stir in lemon juice and fresh parsley.
13. Taste and adjust accordingly.
14. Shift to serving dishes topping each with a drizzle of Private Reserve extra virgin olive oil.
15. Serve and enjoy with couscous or rice.

Easy homemade spaghetti sauce

This is purely a vegetarian spaghetti sauce and can be made ahead of time.

Ingredients

- Bit of dried oregano
- Torn basil and chopped fresh parsley
- 1 medium sized onion
- pinch of sweet paprika
- 4 garlic cloves, minced.
- 2 carrots
- Extra virgin olive oil
- A large 28-ounce can of crushed tomatoes

Directions

1. In a pot, add 2 tablespoons of extra virgin olive oil.
2. Heat over medium temperature until shimmering without smoke.
3. Add chopped onions together with the garlic and finely grated carrots.
4. Cook for 5 minutes while stirring frequently.

5. Add in crushed tomatoes to the mixture with some bit of water.
6. Season with kosher salt and black pepper accordingly.
7. Stir in dry oregano together with the paprika, basil, and parsley.
8. Bring to a boil briefly, then reduce heat.
9. Cover with a lid to simmer for 20 minutes.
10. To let the pasta, absorb some flavors, cover and leave for 6 minutes.
11. Serve and enjoy.

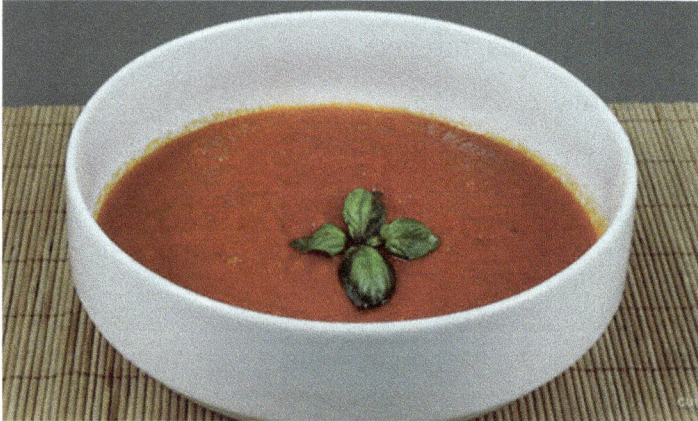

Simple Mediterranean olive oil pasta

The simple Mediterranean olive pasta was inspired by a great Naples dish known as spaghetti aglio e olio where spaghetti in coated by flavorful garlic and oil. It can also be garnished by parsley.

Ingredients

- 6 ounces of marinated artichoke hearts, drained
- ¼ cup of crumbled feta cheese
- 4 garlic cloves, crushed
- Crushed red pepper flakes,
- Salt
- 12 ounces of grape tomatoes, halved
- 15 fresh basil leaves, torn
- ½ cup of early harvest Greek extra virgin olive oil
- 3 scallions
- 1 teaspoon of black pepper
- ¼ cup of pitted olives, halved
- 1 cup of chopped fresh parsley
- 1 lb. thin spaghetti
- Zest of 1 lemon

Directions

1. Cook spaghetti as per the Directions on the package.

2. Drain any excess water and set aside.

3. As the pasta is getting ready, heat the extra virgin olive oil in a large cast iron skillet over medium heat.

4. Lower the heat and add garlic together with a pinch of salt.

5. Let cook briefly, stirring regularly.

6. Stir in the parsley together with the tomatoes and chopped scallions.

7. Cover and continue to cook over low heat until just warmed through, about 30 seconds.

8. Remove from heat, drain any excess cooking water then return to its cooking pot.

9. Pour the warmed olive oil sauce in and toss to coat.

10. Add black pepper and toss.

11. Add the remaining ingredients and toss one more time.

12. Serve and enjoy immediately with feta if you like.

Tahini sauce

If you are looking for a creamy yet rich vegan Mediterranean sauce, then look no further than tahini sauce featuring great flavors and seeds.

Ingredients

- ¾ cup of tahini paste
- 2 garlic cloves
- ½ cup of freshly squeezed lime juice
- 1 cup of fresh chopped parsley leaves
- ½ teaspoon of salt
- ¼ cup of cold water

Directions

1. Crush the garlic cloves with the salt into a paste using a mortar and pestle.
2. Add the crushed garlic with the tahini paste and lime juice to a food processor and blend.
3. Add a little bit of water, continue to blend further until the desired consistency.
4. Shift the tahini to a serving bowl.
5. Serve and enjoy.

Stuffed zucchini boats with tomato and feta

Ingredients

- Kosher salt and pepper
- Splash lemon juice
- Dried oregano
- 6 ounces of cherry tomatoes sliced in halves
- Extra virgin olive oil
- ½ cup of crumbled feta cheese
- 10 fresh mint leaves chopped
- 3 zucchini trimmed and sliced
- Large handful fresh parsley chopped
- Zest of 1 lemon
- 3 green onions both white and green parts, ends trimmed

Directions

1. Heat a cast iron skillet over medium heat.
2. Brush zucchini with extra virgin olive oil on both sides.
3. Season fleshy zucchini side with salt, freshly ground pepper, and oregano.
4. Place zucchini on the preheated grill.

5. Grill for 5 minutes until soft, then turn on back side, also grill for 5 minutes until all sides are tender with some color.
6. Remove zucchini from heat and let cool to handle.
7. With a small spoon, scoop out.
8. Squeeze the liquid out of zucchini flesh.
9. Put the zucchini flesh in a mixing bowl.
10. Add cherry tomatoes together with the green onions, parsley, feta, mint, and lemon zest to the bowl.
11. Add a small splash of lemon juice and sprinkle some oregano.
12. Drizzle a little extra virgin olive oil and mix.
13. Spoon the filling mixture into the prepared zucchini boats and arrange on a serving platter.
14. Serve and enjoy.

Harira recipe

This is a classic Moroccan style lentil and chickpea Mediterranean Sea diet recipe with a full load of warm spices with a vegetarian soup.

Ingredients

- Kosher salt
- 1 cup of red lentils, rinsed
- 1 ½ teaspoons of black pepper
- Lemon wedges
- 1 large yellow onion finely chopped
- 1 ½ teaspoon of turmeric
- 1 carrot peeled and chopped
- 1 teaspoon of cumin
- ¼ cup of long grain rice, rinsed
- Extra virgin olive oil
- ½ teaspoon of ground ginger
- 2 celery stalks chopped
- 4 garlic cloves minced
- 7 cups of vegetable or chicken stock
- ½ teaspoon of ground cinnamon
- ½ teaspoon of cayenne
- 2 14 ounce cans of crushed tomatoes

- 3 tablespoons of tomato paste
- 1 cup packed chopped fresh cilantro
- 1 cup of green lentils, rinsed
- 1 14 ounces can of chickpea

Directions

1. In a large oven, heat 4 tablespoons of extra virgin olive oil until shimmering without smoke over medium heat.
2. Add the onions together with the celery, and carrots.
3. Season with kosher salt and let cook for 5 minutes, stirring regularly.
4. Add the garlic and spices continue to cook for 2 minutes, stirring regularly.
5. Then, add the cilantro, crushed tomatoes, tomato paste, lentils, and chickpeas.
6. Add a little kosher salt let cook for 5 minutes as you stir.
7. Add the broth then increase the heat.
8. Let it boil for 5 minutes.
9. Lower the heat let simmer for 45 minutes when covered to fully cook the legumes.
10. Stir in the rice and continue to cook for 15.
11. Serve and enjoy with lemon wedges.

Homemade granola recipe with olive oil and tahini

This homemade granola recipe features walnuts and variety of dried fruits and irresistibly flavor and nutritional value.

Ingredients

- ½ cup of extra virgin olive oil
- ¾ cup of shelled pistachios
- ¾ cup of walnuts
- ½ cup of sunflower seed
- 3 tablespoons of raw sesame seeds
- 1 cup of unsweetened coconut flakes
- ½ cup of chopped Medjool dates
- ½ cup of dry cranberries
- ¾ cup of honey warmed up
- ½ teaspoon of cardamom
- ⅔ cup of tahini
- 2 teaspoons of pure vanilla extract
- 2 ½ cups of old-fashioned rolled oats
- ½ cup of packed light brown sugar
- ½ teaspoon of ground cinnamon

Directions

1. Heat the oven to 350°F.
2. In a large mixing dish, combine the oats together with the walnuts, pistachios, sesame seeds, sunflower seed, and coconut flakes.
3. In another separate mixing dish, mix the honey together with the tahini, cinnamon, olive oil, brown sugar, vanilla extract, and cardamom.
4. Pour over the oat mixture and toss to coated.
5. Spread the mixture on a large sheet pan in one single layer.
6. Now, bake in the preheated oven for 45 minutes as you stir every 7 minutes, until the mixture is golden.
7. Remove from heat sauce, let cool completely.
8. Break it up into clusters and mix in the dates and cranberries.
9. Serve and enjoy.

Mediterranean party platter

This recipe is a perfect choice to feed a crowd with a healthy Mediterranean diet featuring several fruits and vegetables.

Ingredients

- 6 California fresh figs, halved
- 2 baby eggplants, sliced lengthwise
- Salt
- 1 15-ounces can of good quality marinated artichoke hearts
- 1 teaspoon of sumac
- Olive oil
- Traditional creamy hummus
- 3 ounces of prosciutto di Parma
- Pita bread
- 6 ounces of Greek feta cheese, cubed
- Homemade roasted red pepper hummus
- ½ bell pepper
- Homemade Greek tzatziki
- 6 Campari tomatoes, quartered
- 6 Persian cucumbers, sliced into spears
- Pitted Kalamata olives
- 6 ounces of baby mozzarella cheese balls

Directions

1. Begin by placing the eggplant slices on some paper towels and sprinkle with salt.
2. Sweat out any bitterness for 20 minutes. Let pat dry.
3. Preheat the oven to 400°F.
4. Place the eggplant slices on a lightly oiled baking pan.
5. Drizzle generously with olive oil.
6. Let roast for 20 minutes.
7. On a large serving platter, assemble the remaining ingredients.
8. Begin with the two hummus spreads on opposite sides.
9. Place Tzatziki sauce in the cored bell pepper right at the center of the platter.
10. Any remaining ingredients can be assembled accordingly to your liking.
11. Remove the eggplant from oven, sprinkle with 1 teaspoon of sumac .
12. Add the roasted eggplant to the platter.
13. Refrigerated.
14. Serve and enjoy.

Smoked salmon platter

This recipe combines Mediterranean favorite mainly capers, marinated artichoke hearts and caper.

Ingredients

- 5 radishes, thinly sliced into rounds
- Red pepper flakes or Aleppo pepper
- 12 ounces of smoked salmon
- 1 lemon, cut into wedges
- 4 ounces of cream cheese or Labneh
- Kosher salt
- ⅓ cup of marinated artichoke hearts
- 3 ounces of feta cheese, sliced into slabs
- 1 cucumber, thinly sliced into rounds
- 1 bell pepper (any color), thinly sliced into rounds
- 4 eggs, soft boiled
- 1 vine-ripe tomato, thinly sliced into rounds
- ¼ cup of assorted olives
- 1 small red onion, thinly sliced into rounds

Directions

1. Start by boiling the eggs.

2. Bring a saucepan of water to a boil over medium-high heat.

3. Lower the eggs in the boiling water large.

4. Cook for 6 minutes with a gently boil.

5. Move the eggs to a large bowl of iced water to let cool for 2 minutes.

6. Peel and cut the eggs in halves and season with kosher salt and a pinch of red pepper flakes.

7. Place a small bowl of cream cheese in 1/3 of the platter.

8. Place the feta cheese in different corner of the platter.

9. Arrange the salmon together with the cucumbers, bell peppers, artichoke hearts, tomatoes, olives, radish, onions, and lemon wedges around the cheese.

10. Sprinkle a little red pepper flakes.

11. Serve and enjoy with crackers or crostini.

Roasted red pepper hummus

This is a perfect Mediterranean diet twist with a delicious red pepper roast. It features sumac, smoked paprika, garlic and jalapeno.

Ingredients

- 1 lemon, juice of 1 lemon
- 1 jalapeno pepper, sliced in half length wise
- Salt
- 2 cups of cooked chickpeas
- 2 tablespoons of toasted pine nuts
- 4 garlic cloves, chopped
- Extra virgin olive oil
- 1 red bell pepper, seeded
- 5 tablespoons of tahini paste
- 4g of sumac
- ½ teaspoon of to 1 tsp smoked paprika

Directions

1. Preheat your oven to 450°F.
2. Place the red bell pepper strips and jalapeno in a small baking dish.

3. Drizzle generously with olive oil.

4. Place in the preheated oven and bake for 20 minutes until tender.

5. Remove and drain any excess oil.

6. Add the roasted bell peppers and jalapeno together with the chickpeas, garlic, tahini, smoked paprika, sumac, and lemon juice in a large food processor bowl.

7. Drizzle a little extra virgin olive oil.

8. Run the processor until desired creamy paste consistency.

9. Test and adjust accordingly.

10. Run the processor again to combine.

11. Transfer to a serving bowl. Cover and let chill in a fridge.

12. Serve and enjoy topped with roasted red pepper hummus with a little more extra virgin olive oil with a pinch of paprika.

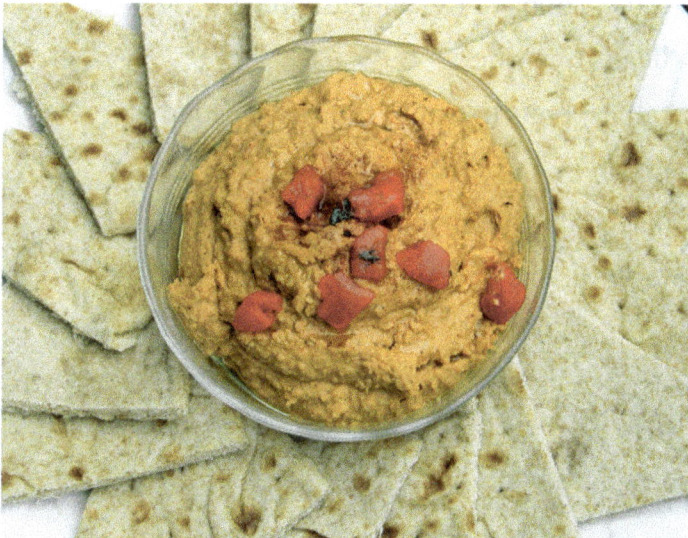

Roasted garlic hummus dip

It is a silky creamy dip very sweet and smoky with enough zing. Feel free to top with pine nuts and feta.

Ingredients

- ½ teaspoon of cayenne pepper
- Private Reserve Greek extra virgin olive oil
- 1 teaspoon of za'atar spice
- 2 ½ cup of cooked chickpeas
- Crumbled feta cheese
- 4 tablespoons of tahini
- Toasted pine nuts
- 3 tablespoons of fresh lemon juice
- 2 heads of garlic
- 2 tablespoons of water, more as needed
- Salt
- 1 teaspoon of sumac
- 3 tablespoons of chopped fresh parsley

Directions

1. Preheat your oven to 400°F.

2. Place the garlic cloves each in a piece of foil that's large enough to wrap around.
3. Lightly drizzle with olive oil.
4. Close the foil up.
5. Bake in the preheated oven for 45 minutes or until the garlic is soft.
6. Remove from heat and let cool briefly, then peel.
7. In the bowl of a food processor, fitted with a blade, place the roasted garlic, chickpeas, lemon juice, tahini, and water.
8. Sprinkle salt, sumac and cayenne.
9. Then, blend until smooth, you can water if dry.
10. Taste and adjust accordingly.
11. Spread the roasted garlic hummus in a bowl.
12. Add a generous drizzle of quality extra virgin olive oil.
13. Top with za'atar spice or parsley, toasted pine nuts, and crumbled feta if desired.
14. Serve with warm pita bread and enjoy.

Antipasto skewers

This recipe is another vegetable blast of a Mediterranean diet. It features marinated vegetables and herbs with festive appetizers to pull the crowd.

Ingredients

- 10 pitted Kalamata olives
- 10 mini wooden skewers
-   • Drizzle extra virgin olive oil
- 20 flat-leaf parsley
- 10 pieces of preserved artichoke hearts
- 10 cherry tomatoes
- 10 pieces of prosciutto di Parma
- Pinch of dried oregano
- 10 mini mozzarella cheese balls

Directions

1. Soak mini wooden skewers in water for one hour.
2. Make sure to Pat dry.
3. Skewer the antipasto ingredients beginning perhaps with the basil or parsley, followed by the larger pieces like prosciutto or artichoke hearts.

4. Place the Kalamata olive at the very top of the skewer.

5. Arrange skewers on a serving platter.

6. Sprinkle with dried oregano and drizzle of extra virgin olive oil.

7. Serve cold or at room temperature.

8. Enjoy.

Baked rice recipe with jam and nuts

Ingredients

- ⅓ cup of shelled pistachios roughly chopped
- 3 tablespoon of fig jam or honey divided
- 13 ounces of round French brie
- ¼ cup of dried mission figs sliced
- ¼ cup of walnut hearts roughly chopped

Directions

1. Preheat the oven to 375°F.
2. Place the fig jam in a microwave-safe dish.
3. Microwave for 30 seconds to soften.
4. In a small bowl, combine the sliced dried figs with the nuts.
5. Add half of the fig jam and mix well to coat with the nut mixture.
6. Place the round of brie in a small cast iron skillet.
7. Using a knife, coat the brie with the remainder of the jam.
8. Top the brie with the fig and nut mixture.
9. Place the dish on top of a baking sheet.
10. Bake on the middle rack of your heated oven for 15 minutes.

11. Remove from the oven and let the brie settle for 5 minutes.
12. Serve warm and enjoy with favorite crackers.

Lentil and rice with crispy onion

This recipe is flavored with the crispy onions, a strong signature copied to the Mediterranean diet from the eastern dishes. It is similar to the Lebanese rose water and orange blossoms.

Ingredients

- 1 cup of black lentils , sorted and rinsed
- Parsley or parsley flakes
- Black pepper
- Oil for frying
- 4 cups of water, divided
- ¼ cup of private reserve Greek extra virgin olive oil
- 2 large yellow onions, diced
- 1 large yellow onion cut in very thin rings
- 1 teaspoon of kosher salt
- 1 cup of long-grain white rice, soaked in water

Directions

1. Place the lentils in a small saucepan with 2 cups of the water.
2. Boil over high heat
3. Lower the heat let simmer while cover until the lentils are par-boiled for 12 minutes.
4. Remove from heat source, drain any excess water then set aside.
5. In a large pan, heat oil over medium-high heat.
6. Add the diced onions and cook until the onions are dark golden brown for 40 minutes.
7. Sprinkle the onions with a teaspoon of salt as they cook.
8. Add the remaining 2 cups of water.
9. Boil over high heat, and then reduce the heat to low let simmer for 2 minutes.
10. Stir the rice and par-cooked lentils into the onion mixture.
11. Cover and bring back to a boil.
12. Stir in a healthy pinch of salt and the black pepper.
13. Reduce the heat to low, cover to absorb any excess liquid in 20 minutes.
14. Remove from heat.
15. Season with salt and pepper to taste.
16. Serve the Mujadara hot or at room temperature with a drizzle of extra virgin olive oil and parsley garnish, if desired.

17. Enjoy.

Vegan chili with quinoa

This is a huge Mediterranean bold twist with a protein power house featuring two different kind of beans with variety of chopped vegetables and packed with rich refreshing flavors.

Ingredients

- ½ teaspoon of ground allspice
- 1 cup of water
- 1 large lime juice of
- ½ large yellow onion chopped
- 1 teaspoon of ground cumin
- ¼ cup of chopped fresh parsley
- 5 garlic cloves minced
- 2 carrots peeled and chopped
- ½ cup of quinoa uncooked
- ½ large green bell pepper chopped
- 1 16-ounces of chopped tomatoes with juice
- 4 cups of low-sodium vegetable broth
- Greek extra virgin olive oil
- 2 ½ teaspoon of chili powder
- 1 15- ounces of kidney beans drained and rinsed
- 1 teaspoon of sweet paprika
- Salt and pepper

- 1 15- ounces of black beans drained and rinsed
- ½ cup of chopped fresh cilantro
- 1 jalapeno sliced

Directions

1. In a small saucepan, combine quinoa and water.
2. Cook over medium heat for 15 minutes until the water is absorbed.
3. Remove from heat and set aside for later.
4. In large saucepan, heat 2 tablespoon of extra virgin olive oil over medium heat until shimmering without smoke.
5. Add onions, garlic, carrots, and bell peppers.
6. Cook for 4 minutes, tossing regularly to softened.
7. Add tomatoes, broth, and spices.
8. Season with salt and pepper.
9. Bring to a boil.
10. Stir in black beans, kidney beans, and partially-cooked quinoa.
11. Reduce the heat let simmer for 25 minutes.
12. Remove from heat source.
13. Stir in cilantro, parsley, and lemon juice.
14. Transfer to serving bowls, drizzle with early harvest extra virgin olive oil and jalapeno slices.
15. Serve and enjoy.

Easy ratatouille recipe

This a typical classic Mediterranean Sea diet vegetable stew features several vegetables especially eggplants, tomatoes, summer squash, flavorful garlic and onions.

Ingredients

- Private reserve Greek extra virgin olive oil
- Eggs over-easy fried
- 1 medium-sized yellow onion finely chopped
- 1 teaspoon of dried rosemary
- 1 tablespoon of sherry vinegar
- 1 green bell pepper stemmed, seeded
- Crusty bread
- 1 lb. eggplant peeled
- 6 garlic cloves peeled, and minced
- 1 teaspoon of sweet paprika
- 2 lb. of vine ripe tomatoes chopped
- 2 zucchini halved length-wise, then cut into ½ inch pieces
- Kosher salt
- ½ cup of red wine
- 2 springs of fresh thyme
- 1 teaspoon of black pepper

- 1 red bell pepper stemmed, seeded
- 3 tablespoons of chopped fresh basil

Directions

1. Place eggplant pieces in a large colander over your sink.
2. Sprinkle with salt let stay for 20 minutes as the eggplant sweats out its bitterness.
3. Pat dry to remove water.
4. In a large heavy pot, heat 2 tablespoons of extra virgin olive oil over medium heat until shimmering without smoke.
5. Add the onions.
6. Let cook while stirring regularly, until onions turn translucent.
7. Now add the red peppers together with the green peppers, continue to cook for 4 minutes, stir.
8. Add the garlic, zucchini, tomatoes, wine, eggplant, and fresh thyme springs.
9. Stir in black pepper, paprika, and rosemary.
10. Season with kosher salt and adjust accordingly.
11. Raise the heat to medium-high, bring to a boil for 5 minutes, stirring twice.
12. Turn down the heat, then cover and cook over low heat for 20 minutes.
13. Remove the ratatouille from the heat.

14. Taste and adjust seasoning accordingly.
15. Add the sherry vinegar and drizzle with extra virgin olive oil.
16. Top with fresh basil.
17. Transfer the ratatouille to dinner bowls, top each with a fried egg and add crusty bread on the side.
18. Serve and enjoy.

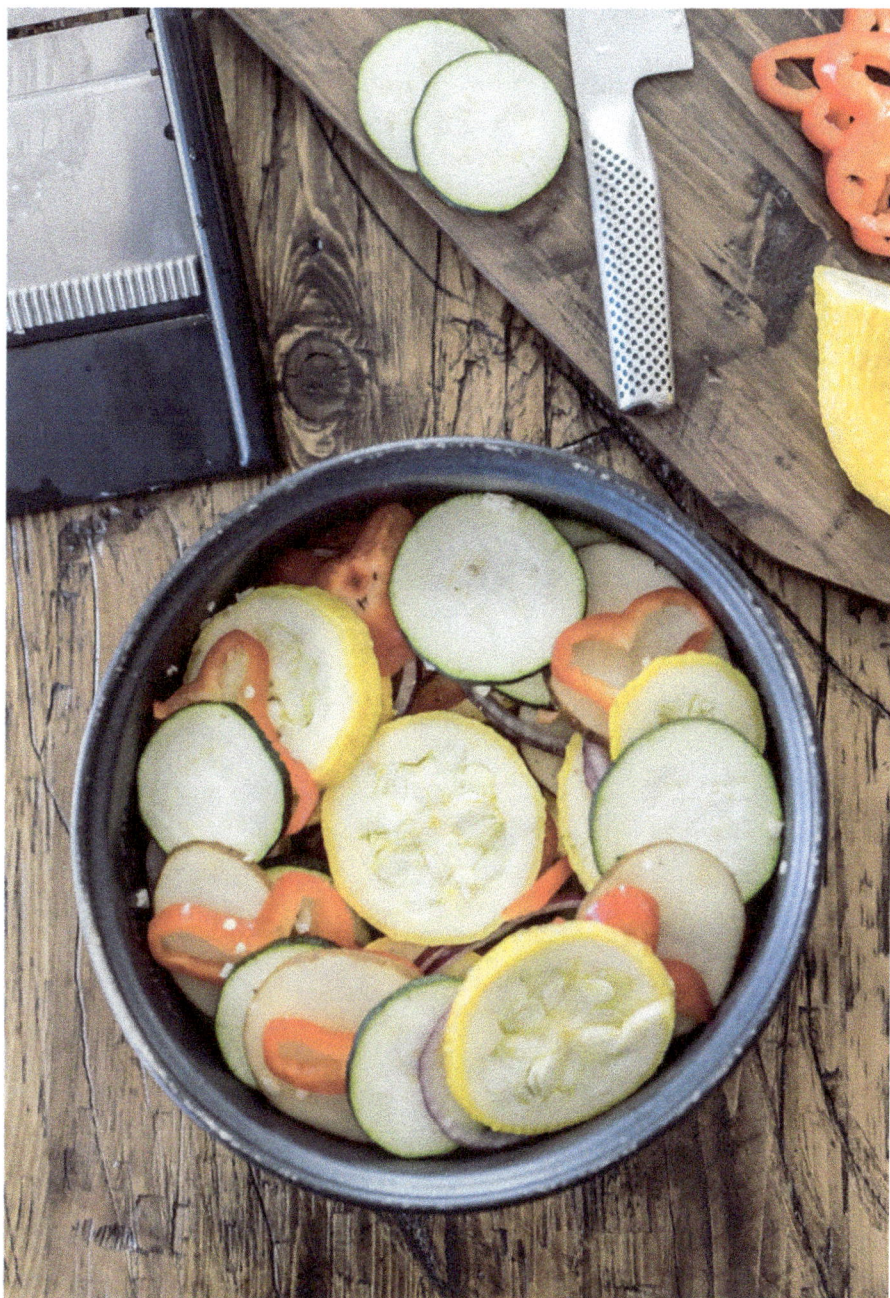

www.ingramcontent.com/pod-product-compliance
Lightning Source LLC
Chambersburg PA
CBHW050747030426
42336CB00012B/1694